Tuina/
Massage
Manipulations

Tuina/ Massage Manipulations

Basic Principles and Techniques

Chief Editor: Li Jiangshan

SINGING
DRAGON

LONDON AND PHILADELPHIA

Chief Translators: Henry A. and Buchtel V.
Assistant Editors: Li Tielang and Zhou Guoping
Editorial Committee: Ai Kun, Peng Liang and Liu Qiong

First published in 2009
by People's Military Medical Press

This edition published in 2011
by Singing Dragon
an imprint of Jessica Kingsley Publishers
in co-operation with People's Military Medical Press
116 Pentonville Road
London N1 9JB, UK
and
400 Market Street, Suite 400
Philadelphia, PA 19106, USA

www.singingdragon.com

Copyright © People's Military Medical Press 2009 and 2011

Library of Congress Cataloging in Publication Data
A CIP catalog record for this book is available from the Library of Congress

British Library Cataloguing in Publication Data
A CIP catalogue record for this book is available from the British Library

ISBN 978 1 84819 058 0

Printed and bound in Great Britain by
MPG Books Group

Contents

Preface

Tuina, based on the theories of Traditional Chinese Medicine, uses specific manipulations or massage tools to operate on certain areas or acupoints on the surface of the body. Tuina treatment can regulate the body's physiological and pathological condition to treat and prevent disease, improve health, and strengthen the body. As manipulations are the primary method of carrying out treatment, they are a core component of the study of Tuina, and are also the most difficult skills to master.

In order to meet the requirements of Tuina education and to simplify communication with international medical massage professionals, this book lays stress on the analysis of the structure of traditional manipulations, as well as the training of clinical skills. Video and text are combined to demonstrate the manipulations, and provide a complete method for learning the basic skills of Tuina and at the same time resolving the issue of how to study further without the direct guidance of a teacher.

This book is divided into two sections: the first introduces the definitions, classifications, and requirements of each Tuina manipulation, as well as common Tuina media; the second describes the main points, cautions, and clinical application of the most common adult manipulations.

During the editing of this book emphasis was placed on the clinical applicability of the manipulation skills, and great care was taken to make the content accurate, the main points and different levels clear, and the writing easy to understand. In spite of this, oversights and shortcomings are unavoidable, and it is hoped that colleagues and readers will offer their valuable criticism and corrections.

CHAPTER 1

Concept of Chinese Tuina Manipulations

Chinese Tuina is an external therapeutic method that is guided both by Traditional Chinese Medical theories and those of modern medicine. It expounds upon and researches the use of manipulation therapy and self-cultivation training to prevent and cure illness. In ancient days, *tui na* (literally meaning push–grasp) was also called *an mo* (press–rub), *an qiao* (press–step), *qiao mo* (step–rub), *jiao yin* (raise–stretch) and *an wu* (press–thrust).

A core component of Chinese Tuina is manipulation therapy. Manipulation therapy is a treatment method in which standardized actions are performed by the practitioner on the surface of the recipient's body using the hands, other parts of the body or specialized tools. The goal is to prevent and cure disease, and the practitioner's level of familiarity with the operation and application of each manipulation directly influences the efficacy of the treatment.

1. Manipulation Classification

There are many ways to classify Chinese Tuina manipulations: according to the morphological characteristics, area of treatment, direction of force, target patient, etc. Currently, most scholars classify manipulations according to the morphological characteristics of the movement. Following the principles of this classification method allows us to divide all of the basic manipulations into the following six categories.

Swinging Manipulations

Manipulations in which action initiated by the forearm causes the wrist joint to perform side-to-side swinging movements are classified as swinging manipulations. Some examples are one-finger pushing meditation, rocking and kneading.

Rubbing Manipulations

Rubbing manipulations include those that involve friction between the practitioner's hand and the surface of the recipient's body. For example, rubbing, scrubbing, pushing and twisting.

Vibrating Manipulations

In this category of manipulations specific muscular activity on the part of the practitioner creates an obvious sensation of vibration in the subcutaneous tissue of the recipient. Examples include vibration and shaking.

Compression Manipulations

In this category pressure is applied vertically onto or from both sides of a certain area. It includes pressing, digital pressing, squeezing, grasping, finger twisting and plucking.

Striking Manipulations

Striking manipulations are those that involve rhythmic striking of the surface of the recipient's body. Patting, striking and tapping are included in this category.

Joint Manipulation Techniques

In this class of manipulations the practitioner uses certain techniques to passively manipulate the recipient's joints within their normal physiological range. It includes swinging, thrusting and counter-traction.

2. Requirements of Tuina

In order to achieve the desired penetrating effect, Tuina manipulations must be performed in accordance with basic requirements regarding duration, strength, uniformity and gentleness.

Duration

Each manipulation must be performed for a specified period of time without loss of quality in order to preserve the continuity of the movement.

Strength

The manipulations must possess a certain degree of power, effect and dexterity.

Uniformity

The manipulations must be rhythmic, and should not alternate between fast and slow. In addition, in most situations the manipulations should be performed with a steady level of force, and should not suddenly get lighter or heavier.

Gentleness

The manipulation should be done with an appropriate level of strength and should morph into other manipulations naturally and smoothly.

Penetration

The effect of the manipulation should penetrate to the area of pathology.

3. Tuina Media

During a Tuina treatment various liquids, pastes or powders can be applied to the skin to reduce friction or to obtain a certain medicinal effect. These materials are called Tuina media. The most frequently used media are as follows.

Talcum Powder

Talcum powder has the effect of lubricating the skin. It is often used in the summer and can be used during the treatment of various disease patterns.

Baby Powder

Baby powder has the effects of lubricating the skin and absorbing sweat and moisture. It can be used for various kinds of disease patterns.

Onion-Ginger Juice

Onion-ginger juice can be extracted by mashing up onion stems and fresh ginger or by soaking sliced onion stems and fresh ginger in 75% alcohol. It can strengthen the effects of warming and dispersing cold; it is often used in winter and spring and when treating children with deficiency cold syndrome.

Rice Liquor

This potable liquor has the effects of activating blood, expelling pathogenic wind, dissipating cold, eliminating dampness, unblocking the meridians and freeing the collaterals. It can be used to reduce fever and is indicated in cases of acute sprain.

Wintergreen Ointment

This ointment is a combination of wintergreen oil, menthol, Vaseline (petroleum jelly) and a small amount of musk. It has the therapeutic effects of warming the meridians to dissipate cold and lubricating the skin. It is indicated for children with deficiency cold diarrhoea and soft tissue injuries.

Mint Juice

Mint juice is made by mixing 5g of 5% menthol with 100ml of 75% alcohol. It has the effects of warming meridians to dissipate cold, releasing the exterior by cooling, clearing and relieving the head and eyes and lubricating the skin. It is indicated for children with deficiency cold diarrhoea and soft tissue injuries. It can be used in conjunction with scrubbing or press-kneading to strengthen the penetrating heat effect.

Water

Cool and clean potable water has the effects of cooling the skin and reducing fever, and is indicated for externally contracted heat patterns.

Safflower Oil

Safflower oil for this purpose is made up with wintergreen oil, safflower, and menthol. It has the therapeutic effects of reducing swelling and relieving pain and is often used in the treatment of acute or chronic soft tissue injuries.

Sesame Oil

This refers to edible sesame oil. When performing the scrubbing manipulation, daubing some sesame oil on the skin can assist with heat penetration to raise the efficacy of the treatment. It is often used when performing scraping (*gua sha*).

Egg White

Remove the egg white by making a hole in the egg. It has the effects of clearing and cooling heat and removing food accumulation. It is used in the treatment of fever induced by external pathogens and poor digestion.

CHAPTER 2

Swinging Manipulations

Swinging manipulations involve coordinated and continuous swinging of the fingers, palms or wrist joint. This category of manipulations is primarily composed of one-finger pushing meditation, rolling and kneading.

1. One-Finger Pushing Meditation

In one-finger pushing meditation force is exerted through the tip or pad of the thumb. The thumb joint flexes and extends, driven by the back and forth swaying of the wrist joint, and force is transmitted through the thumb to act continuously upon the treatment area or acupoint. One-finger pushing meditation is the representative manipulation of the one-finger pushing meditation school. The movement is difficult and stresses the use of internal force.

Movement Principles

POSTURE

The word *relaxed* defines the movement from beginning to finish. The shoulders and arms are relaxed and sunken; do not shrug or lift the shoulders. The wrist is flexed naturally; do not stiffen the joint or use force. With the exception of the thumb, the fingers and palm are relaxed and do not use force. The tip or pad of the thumb adheres firmly to a certain point and does not leave the skin or rub back and forth along the surface. (Fig. 1)

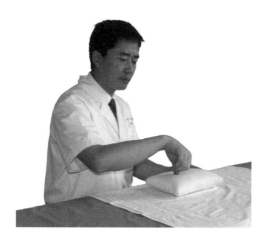

Fig. 1 Practicing posture of one-finger pushing meditation

BASIC MOVEMENT

With the elbow area acting as a pivot, swinging is initiated by the forearm, which in turn drives the swinging of the wrist. If the range of movement of the practitioner's interphalangeal thumb joints is relatively small or if mild stimulation is called for, the swinging of the wrist may in turn drive the flexion and extension of the interphalangeal joints of the thumb. (Fig. 2)

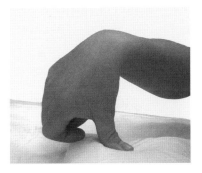

Fig. 2A Wrist rotates outward and thumb extends

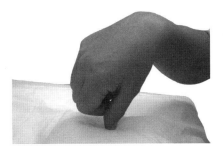

Fig. 2B Wrist rotates inward and thumb contracts

Fig. 2 Basic movement of one-finger pushing meditation

SWING QUICKLY AND MOVE SLOWLY

The swinging motion is performed quickly (usually about 120–160 times per minute) while the movement along the surface of the body is slow.

Cautions

During the operation one's attention should be focused.

Do not bend your back, raise your shoulders, stick out your elbows, or stiffen the wrist joint.

Rubbing, sliding and hopping should not occur at the area of contact.

Clinical Application

One-finger pushing meditation provides moderate stimulation with great penetrating force on a small contact area. It can be used on meridians and points all over the body, and is often used in the treatment of internal medicine disease patterns such as headache, dizziness, cough, epigastric pain and abdominal pain.

Variations

THUMB SIDE PUSHING MEDITATION

In this variation force is exerted through the radial side of the thumb. The swaying is initiated by the forearm, which drives the back and forth swinging of the wrist, which in turn flexes and extends the thumb joint. The basic requirements of this manipulation include sunken shoulders, hanging elbows, level wrist, empty palm and firm thumb, and the swinging motion is repeated 120–160 times per minute. This variation provides relatively gentle stimulation, so it is used primarily on the facial area, head, chest and abdomen. It is applied in the treatment of internal medicine diseases such as facial paralysis, near-sightedness, insomnia, headache and diarrhoea. (Fig. 3)

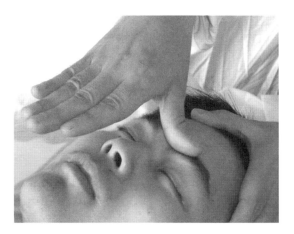

Fig. 3 Thumb side pushing meditation

BENT THUMB PUSHING MEDITATION

In this method the radial side of the back of the interphalangeal thumb joint is used to contact the treatment area. Active swinging of the forearm drives the continuous flexion and extension of the wrist joint. The characteristics of bent thumb pushing meditation are that the exertion of force is stable, it 'sticks' to the surface well, and is powerful and vigorous. It can be on the nape and neck areas, on suture joint areas and on the soles of the feet. (Fig. 4)

TWINING

Twining makes use of either the radial side of the thumb or the tip of the thumb as above, but the swinging motion is performed faster (over 200 times per minute). In this manipulation the frequency of the swinging motion of the wrist is high and the stimulation is moderate. This method is most often applied on areas of pathological change as it has the effects of softening hardness, dissipating accumulation and swelling and relieving pain. It is applicable in the case of the external medicine carbuncle, swelling, sore and furuncle diseases such as mastitis, swollen and sore throat, clove sore and swollen boil.

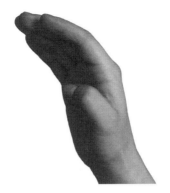

Fig. 4A

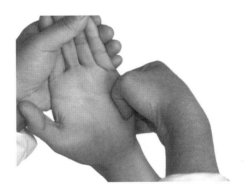

Fig. 4B

Fig. 4 Bent thumb pushing meditation

2. Rocking

The term rocking has both a general and specific usage. Specifically, it refers to a manipulation in which the practitioner forms a hollow fist and places the knuckle of the first interphalangeal joint of the index, middle, ring and little fingers on the treatment area. A swinging motion is initiated by the forearm, causing the wrist to flex and extend, rocking the back of the fist back and forth on the surface of the body. Generally, the term is also used to refer collectively to rocking, rolling and forearm rolling. Rocking is a supportive manipulation used by the one-finger pushing meditation school. (Fig. 5)

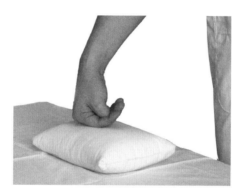

Fig. 5 Rocking

Movement Principles

POSTURE

The shoulder and arm are relaxed, the elbow joint is flexed to an angle of 160° and the hand is formed into a hollow fist.

BASIC MOVEMENT

The swinging motion of the forearm causes flexion and extension of the wrist. The range of the rocking motion is kept within about 90°, meaning that the forward and backward motions of the fist are each about 45°.

ROCK FAST AND MOVE SLOW

The rate of rocking should be fast (between 120–160 times per minute) and the movement along the surface of the recipient's body should be slow.

Cautions

The index, middle, ring and little fingers should be flexed naturally and not pinched together.

While rocking do not leave or rub the surface of the skin.

Clinical Application

Rocking manipulation has a relatively large contact area and can provide moderate to strong stimulation. It is usually used on the head, nape and neck area, shoulder and upper back area, lower back and heavily-muscled areas of the limbs. It is used in the treatment of headache, sequelae of stroke, lower back muscle strain, cervical spine pathology, etc.

3. Rolling

The practitioner uses the ulnar side (little finger side) of the back of the hand to exert force on a certain area. The combination of rotating the forearm and flexing and extending the wrist causes the *little fish side* (hypothenar eminence) and fingers to roll back and forth continuously on the treatment area. (Fig. 6) This method is the representative therapeutic manipulation of the rolling school of Tuina.

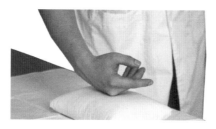

Fig. 6 Rolling

Movement Principles

POSTURE

Sink and relax the shoulders and arms and flex the elbow at an angle of 120–140°. Relax the hand and wrist. Flex the metacarpophalangeal joints naturally, and allow the fingers to spread out and come together naturally as they roll. (Fig. 7)

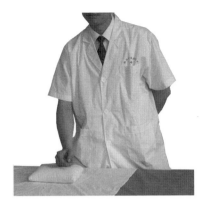

Fig. 7A

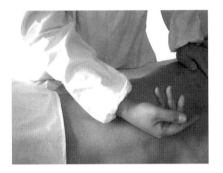

Fig. 7B

Fig. 7 Posture of rolling

BASIC MOVEMENT

As the forearm rotates out (supination) the wrist joint flexes, and as the forearm rotates in (pronation) the wrist extends.

RANGE OF MOTION

The range of the rolling motion is kept to about 120°; as the wrist flexes the hand rolls outward to about 80° and as the wrist extends the hand rolls inward to about 40°.

FORWARD THREE, RETURN ONE

The pressure applied when rolling forward is 3 times that of when rolling back, therefore a ratio of 3:1.

ROLL FAST AND MOVE SLOW

The frequency of the rolling is relatively fast (about 140 times per minute) and the movement along the body surface is slow.

Cautions

Scrubbing, striking, dragging or jumping along the body surface is not allowed.

The movements should be soft and gentle. Avoid using sudden force as it will cause a sensation of being struck.

Clinical Application

The contact area of rolling manipulation is relatively diffuse and the pressure is heavy, providing moderate and comfortable stimulation. It can be used on the nape of the neck, shoulders, upper back, lower back and buttocks, as well as on heavily-muscled areas of the limbs. It is often combined with joint manipulation techniques to treat diseases of the musculoskeletal and nervous systems such as impediment pattern, wilting pattern, sequelae of stroke, stiff neck, prolapse of the lumbar intervertebral disc, periarthritis of the shoulder and cervical spine pathology.

Variations

KNUCKLE ROLLING

The practitioner exerts force through the back side of the metacarpophalangeal joints of the middle, ring and little fingers. The movement principles are basically the same as those for rocking. During the operation, the range of flexion and extension of the wrist joint is less than in rocking, but the force applied is stronger. It is generally used on heavily-muscled areas of the body.

FOREARM ROLLING

In this variation swinging is initiated by the upper arm, causing the ulnar side of the forearm to roll back and forth and exert force on the treatment area. The movement principles are basically the same as those for rocking. It is generally used on heavily-muscled areas of the body.

4. Kneading

In this manipulation the *big fish side* (thenar eminence), heel of the palm, forearm or finger pads are placed firmly on a certain area or acupoint and are used to perform light and gentle circular motions that knead both the skin and the tissue beneath it. (Fig. 8)

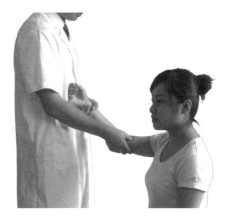

Fig. 8 Kneading

Movement Principles

POSTURE

Relax the shoulders, forearm and wrist.

BASIC MOVEMENT

Back and forth movements initiated by the forearm drive the wrist, palm or finger pads to make light and gentle circular motions that move the subcutaneous tissues.

The manipulations should be soft and rhythmic throughout, starting with a small range of motion and slowly increasing.

SPECIFIC OPERATION

- **Finger kneading.** Finger kneading is done with the pads of the thumb, the middle finger, or the index, middle and ring fingers together. The movement is initiated by the forearm, which drives the wrist and the finger pads to perform light, soft and gentle circular motions. The movement frequency is between 120–160 times per minute. (Fig. 9)

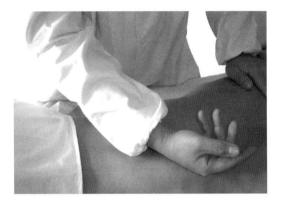

Fig. 9 Finger kneading

- **Palm kneading.** Palm kneading can be done using the palm, the base of the palm or the *big fish side*. The forearm connects with the wrist to carry out the circular kneading movement. (Fig. 10)

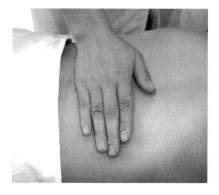

Fig. 10 Palm kneading

- **Forearm kneading.** Small circular movements are initiated by the shoulder joint and drive the heavily-muscled area of the ulnar side (little finger side) of the forearm to perform circular kneading on the treatment area. (Fig. 11)

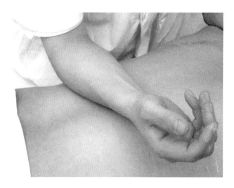

Fig. 11 Forearm kneading

Cautions

While performing the manipulation the area of contact must be firm to prevent rubbing or sliding along the surface of the body.

The movements should be gentle; hard pressing is not allowed.

Clinical Application

As this manipulation is light, soft and gentle and provides a low level of stimulation, it is commonly used in relaxation or health cultivation massage manipulation. Finger kneading can be used along any meridian or acupoint. Palm kneading can be applied to the head, face, chest, abdomen, lumbosacral area and limbs. Forearm kneading is used on the lower and upper back, buttocks and heavily-muscled areas. Kneading can be used in the treatment of many different disease patterns, including poor digestion, headache, dizziness, soft-tissue injury, tinnitus and impotence.

CHAPTER 3

Rubbing Manipulations

These manipulations are performed by making circular or back and forth movements using the fingers, palm and elbow on the surface of the body. They include pushing, rubbing, scrubbing, twisting and scraping.

1. Pushing

This manipulation is performed by making a straight pushing movement in one direction on a certain part of the body or acupoint using the fingers, palm or elbow. (Fig. 12)

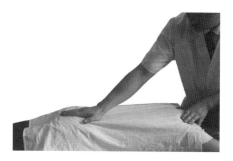

Fig. 12 Pushing

Movement Principles

While pushing, the fingers, palm or elbow should press firmly on the skin with even pressure. The pushing should be done slowly.

Tuina media such as safflower oil, talcum powder or massage oil may be used to prevent injury to the skin.

SPECIFIC OPERATION

- **Finger pushing.** Pushing along a meridian or parallel to the muscle fibres with the pad of the thumb or middle finger.

- **Palm pushing.** Pushing in a straight line with the palm. (Fig. 13)

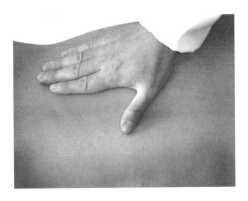

Fig. 13 Palm pushing

- **Elbow pushing**. Pushing in a certain direction with the tip of the elbow (the olecranon process of the ulna) when the elbow joint is flexed. (Fig. 14)

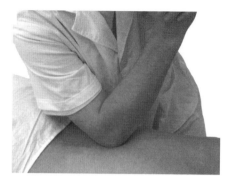

Fig. 14 Elbow pushing

Cautions

Pushing is done in a straight line in a single direction; it should not be used to perform curved lines.

Do not use great force or heavy pressure so as to avoid injuring the skin.

Clinical Application

Pushing manipulation is gentle and soothing and provides a moderate level of stimulation. It has the effect of unblocking meridians, activating the collaterals and dissipating blood stasis and accumulation, and is a very common clinical manipulation. Finger pushing has a small contact area and short range of motion, so it is frequently employed on the face and hands. Palm pushing has a larger contact area and longer range, so it is frequently applied to the upper and lower back, chest, abdomen and limbs. The pressure provided by elbow pushing is relatively strong, so it is used along the spine and on the back of the thigh. Pushing is often used in the treatment of disease patterns such as cold, wind and damp impediment pain, rigidity of the neck, heat effusion, muscle spasm, and chest and rib-side distension and pain.

2. Rubbing

The forearm and wrist move together to produce circular rhythmic stroking motions on the surface of the body with the finger pads or palm. (Fig. 15)

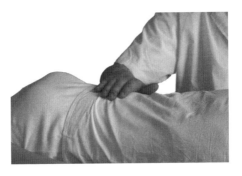

Fig. 15 Rubbing

Movement Principles

POSTURE

With the shoulders, elbow and wrist relaxed, slightly flex the elbow and place the finger pads or palm on the surface of the skin.

BASIC MOVEMENT

The forearm and wrist move together to produce gentle, harmonious circular stroking motions.

The movement can be performed clockwise or anti-clockwise, and should be performed at a rate of 120 times per minute.

Cautions

Use light force and avoid moving the subcutaneous tissue.

Clinical Application

As the stimulation provided by rubbing is light, gentle and harmonious, it is a common manipulation in health cultivation massage. Finger rubbing is most often applied to the face; palm rubbing is appropriate for use on the chest, abdomen and ribs. Rubbing is often used in the treatment of disease patterns such as abdominal distension, diarrhoea, constipation, intestinal disorder, abnormal menstruation, menstrual pain and insomnia.

3. Scrubbing

Scrubbing refers to light back and forth rubbing performed on the surface of the body using the palm, *big fish side* (thenar eminence) or *little fish side* (hypothenar eminence). (Fig. 16–18)

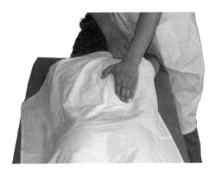

Fig. 16 Scrubbing

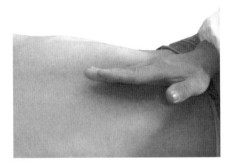

Fig. 17 Little fish side scrubbing

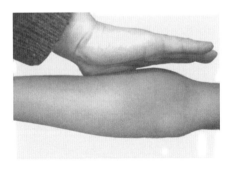

Fig. 18 Big fish side scrubbing

Movement Principles

Breathe naturally, keep the shoulders relaxed and extend the wrist naturally.

The back and forth rubbing movements should be fast, even, long and straight.

Rubbing should be performed on exposed skin, so use lubricating media (such as Chinese ilex paste or sesame oil) if necessary, to avoid skin abrasion.

Cautions

Breathe naturally and do not hold your breath.

Do not use too much force so as to avoid injury to the skin.

Clinical Application

This manipulation provides heavy stimulation and has a powerful effect in warming the meridians and dissipating cold. After application of this manipulation the blood vessels of the contact area are dilated and the skin is reddened, so it is often used as a closing manipulation for a treatment. Palm scrubbing is usually used on large smooth areas such as the chest, rib-sides, abdomen, shoulders and upper back. *Big fish side* scrubbing is usually used on the upper limbs. *Little fish side* scrubbing has a relatively small contact area, so it is usually used on the lumbosacral area, either side of the spine, and the shoulders and upper back. Scrubbing is used in the treatment of disease patterns such as abdominal pain or diarrhoea caused by spleen and stomach vacuity and cold, and urinal incontinence, impotence, and gynecological disease caused by spleen and kidney yang vacuity. It can also be used to treat wind damp impediment pain, soft tissue injury, swelling and pain, and reduced joint mobility.

4. Twisting

Twisting is a manipulation performed by clasping a certain area of the body with both palms and moving the hands in opposite directions to twist and knead while simultaneously moving up and down along the limb. (Fig. 19–21)

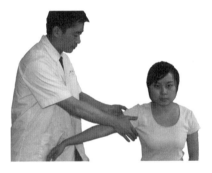

Fig. 19 Upper limb twisting

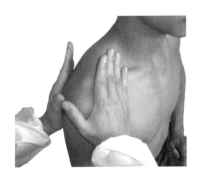

Fig. 20 Shoulder twisting

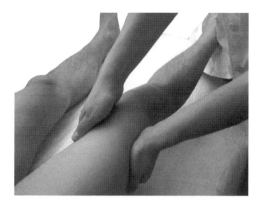

Fig. 21 Lower limb twisting

Movement Principles

POSTURE

Relax the shoulders, extend the hands naturally and keep the palms empty.

BASIC MOVEMENT

With the shoulders as acting as a pivot, the upper arms drive the flexion and contraction of the elbows, causing the palms to twist as if twisting up a hemp rope.

With the hands pressing towards each other, twist quickly and move up or down slowly.

Cautions

The practitioner should breathe naturally and avoid holding their breath.

The twisting should be continuous; there should be no breaks or pauses in the movement.

Clinical Application

Twisting is a supportive manipulation with a relatively gentle stimulation. It has the effects of relaxing the muscles and relieving weariness, so it is frequently combined with shaking and used to end a Tuina treatment session. It is appropriate for use on the lower back, upper back, ribs and limbs, especially the upper limbs. It is often applied in the treatment of sinew injuries of limb joints, back pain, rib-side distension and pain, etc.

5. Scraping

The radial side of the thumb or the pads of the index and middle fingers are first dipped in water and then are used to push rapidly in one direction on a certain area or acupoint. (Fig. 22)

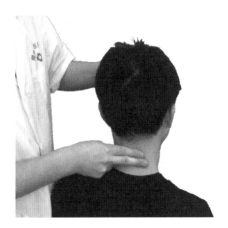

Fig. 22 Scraping

Movement Principles

The movements should be dexterous and quick. Stop when purplish-red macules appear on the treatment area to avoid injuring the skin.

Tuina media such as water, sesame oil or onion-ginger juice can be used during the operation to prevent injury to the skin.

Specialized tools such as scraping boards (*gua sha ban*) and soup spoons (*tang shao*) may also be used.

Cautions

Movements should be dexterous and quick, and injury to the skin should be avoided.

Clinical Application

Scraping (*gua sha*) provides moderate stimulation and has the effects of expelling wind, dispelling cold, descending qi and arresting vomit. It is frequently used on the neck, shoulders, chest, ribs and along the thoracic spine, and is used in the treatment of disease patterns such as summerheat heat, vomiting, externally contracted heat effusion and rigid neck.

CHAPTER 4

Vibration Manipulations

The manipulations in this category involve rhythmic alternation between heavy and light high-frequency rhythmic stimulation. They include shaking and vibrating.

1. Shaking

The practitioner holds the distal end of the recipient's limbs with a single hand or both hands and performs constant, limited-range, high-frequency, up–down or left–right shaking, providing a feeling of loose motion in the joints and muscles. This category includes arm shaking and leg shaking.

Movement Principles

POSTURE

Breathe naturally and grasp the distal end of the recipient's limb with one or both hands using an appropriate amount of force.

BASIC MOVEMENT

The upper arm initiates movement, causing the wrist to perform small-range up–down or side-to-side shaking.

Although the range of motion is small, the frequency of the shaking should be fast; shaking the upper limbs can be done at 200 times per minute and the lower limbs can be done at 100 times per minute.

SPECIFIC OPERATION

- **Arm shaking.** The recipient sits or lies down with their shoulders and arms relaxed. The practitioner stands to the front and to one side, or at the recipient's side, then leans forward slightly and holds the recipient's wrist with two hands or holds the distal end of the recipient's arm with a single hand. The arm is slowly raised up to the front-side to an angle of about 60° and then is shaken continuously sideways or up and down. (Fig. 23)

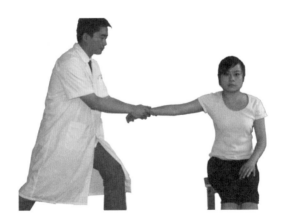

Fig. 23 Arm shaking

- **Leg shaking.** The recipient lies on their back with their lower limbs relaxed. The practitioner stands behind the recipient's feet and holds one ankle with each hand. The legs are raised to an angle of about 15–30° and then are shaken up and down. (Fig. 24)

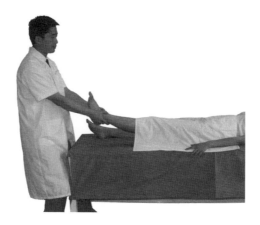

Fig. 24 Leg shaking

Cautions

The practitioner should continue to breathe naturally and avoid holding their breath.

Excessive force should not be used when grasping both of the recipient's hands to avoid making the movements too hard.

Clinical Application

Shaking is a gentle, light and fast manipulation, and has the effects of soothing and enlivening sinews and collaterals and lubricating the joints. This manipulation is often combined with twisting to end a treatment session. It is used on the limbs in the treatment of disease patterns such as periarthritis of the shoulder, acute lumbar sprain and prolapse of the lumbar intervertebral disc.

2. Vibrating

The fingers or palm are placed firmly on a certain area and high-frequency, limited-range vibrations are performed. This manipulation is also called trembling (*zhen chan*), and it includes finger vibrating and palm vibrating. (Fig. 25)

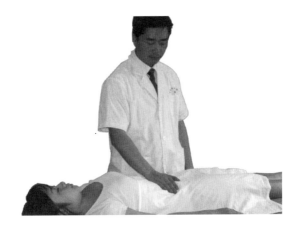

Fig. 25 Vibrating

Movement Principles

POSTURE

Breathe naturally. Place the fingers or palm firmly on the surface of the skin.

BASIC MOVEMENT

Static use of force by the forearm causes a sensation of vibration to be transmitted continuously into the recipient's body.

The movements are continuous and connected. The frequency of the vibration should be 400 times per minute or more.

SPECIFIC OPERATION

- **Finger vibrating.** The practitioner places either the thumb or the middle finger or the thumb and index fingers together firmly onto meridians and acupoints. The muscles of the forearm are contracted powerfully and static force is used to create intense vibration that is concentrated into the tips of the fingers and transmitted into the recipient's body.

- **Palm vibrating.** A single palm or stacked palms are placed on an area of the recipient's body or clasp both sides of a limb and vibrate.

Cautions

The practitioner should breathe naturally and should not hold their breath.

Do not use a large amount of pressure, and avoid stopping and starting.

Clinical Application

Vibration is the representative manipulation of the internal-cultivation school of Tuina. This manipulation has the effects of warming, supplementing and regulating, and is often used on patients with yang qi vacuity and blocked channels and collaterals. Finger vibration is applicable to acupoints over the entire body; palm vibration is most often used on the epigastric region, abdomen, waist and back. Vibration can be used in the treatment of headache, insomnia, distension and pain of the epigastric region and poor digestion.

CHAPTER 5

Compression Manipulations

Compression manipulations are performed using the fingers, palms or other parts of the limbs to press or squeeze the treatment area. It comprises more than ten separate manipulations, including pressing, digital pressing, nipping, squeezing, grasping, plucking, finger twisting and sliding.

1. Pressing

The practitioner uses the fingers, palm or elbow to gradually apply and maintain pressure on a certain part of the body or acupoint. (Fig. 26–29)

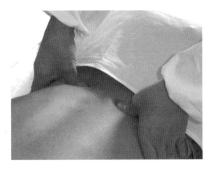

Fig. 26 Finger pressing

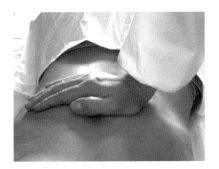

Fig. 27 Single-palm pressing

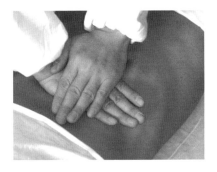

Fig. 28 Stacked-palm pressing

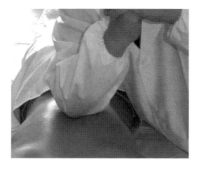

Fig. 29 Elbow pressing

Movement Principles

Force should be exerted vertically on the body surface. The pressure starts light and steadily gets heavier until the area receiving pressure 'obtains qi' (*de qi*); namely obtaining sensations of soreness, distension, warmth and numbness.

When finishing the manipulation the pressure should be released gradually and kneading may be done at the same time.

Cautions

There should be a firm connection between the area exerting force and the surface of the body and there should be no horizontal movement.

Neither sudden use of force nor excessive pressure is allowed.

Clinical Application

Pressing provides a strong stimulation and is also very comfortable. It is one of the most ancient Tuina manipulations. Finger pressing can be used on any area or acupoint; palm pressing is usually used on wide and flat areas such as the lower and upper back, chest and abdomen; elbow pressing is appropriate for use on the buttocks, lumbosacral area, etc. Pressing can be applied in the treatment of a variety of disease patterns such as diarrhoea, headache, epigastric region pain, soreness and numbness of the limbs, soft tissue injury and functional scoliosis.

2. Digital Pressing

The tip of the thumb or the middle knuckles (flexed proximal interphalangeal joints) of the thumb, index and middle fingers are used to press on acupoints or on specific areas. (Fig. 30)

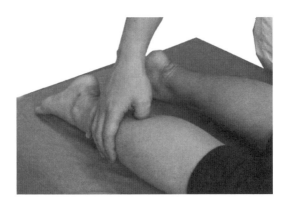

Fig. 30 Digital pressing

Movement Principles

Force should be applied directly downward on the surface of the body. It starts light and gradually gets heavier, producing quite strong sensations of soreness and distension in the treatment area.

Digital pressing may be followed by press-kneading to relieve localized discomfort.

SPECIFIC OPERATION

- **Thumb tip digital pressing.** First make a loose fist, then straighten the thumb and place it close to the side of the index finger (second phalanges). The tip of the thumb is used to apply pressure.

- **Thumb knuckle digital pressing.** The thumb is flexed and the radial side of the middle knuckle (metacarpophalangeal joint) of the thumb is used to apply pressure. For extra support, the tip of the thumb may be placed on the outer border of the index finger (second phalanges). (Fig. 31)

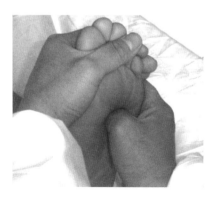

Fig. 31 Thumb knuckle digital pressing

- **Index knuckle digital pressing.** With the index finger flexed, form a fist with the other fingers and use the middle joint of the index finger (proximal interphalangeal joint) to apply pressure. For extra support, the inner border of the last joint of the thumb may be pressed tightly to the fingernail of the index finger. (Fig. 32)

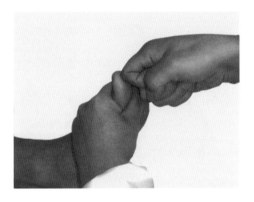

Fig. 32 Index knuckle digital pressing

Cautions

When pressing, the point of contact should be firm and there should be no movement along the surface of the body.

Sudden or violent use of force is prohibited.

Clinical Application

Digital pressing provides strong stimulation and has a relatively powerful effect in unblocking meridians and relieving pain. It is quite effective in the treatment of various pain-related diseases. This manipulation can be used on acupoints all over the body, as well as the inner side of joints of the limbs. It is used in the treatment of various pain patterns.

3. Nipping

The thumbnail is used to press vertically on and sharply stimulate a certain area or acupoint. (Fig. 33)

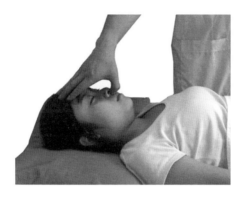

Fig. 33 Nipping

Movement Principles

POSTURE

Relax the shoulders and arms, straighten the thumb and focus strength on the fingertip.

The exertion of force should be vertical and steady, and should move from light to heavy. Make sure the force penetrates deeply. After nipping, lightly knead the treatment area to relieve discomfort.

The manipulation should be performed about 4 to 5 times and stopped when the symptoms show improvement.

When used as a part of emergency first aid, the manipulation should be strong and quick and the number of repetitions should be limited.

Cautions

The fingernail used should not be overly long in order to prevent injury to the skin.

Clinical Application

Nipping provides strong stimulation and has the effects of opening the orifices (to induce resuscitation), settling fright and relieving pain. The method is usually used on acupoints of the face and limbs and is used most frequently in emergency first aid.

4. Squeezing

The thumb pad is used in opposition to the pads of the index and middle fingers (or in opposition to the other four fingers) to repeatedly squeeze and release the skin. (Fig. 34)

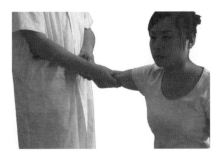

Fig. 34 Squeezing

Movement Principles

The finger pads are used in opposition to each other to squeeze, immediately release, and then squeeze again, combined with movement along the body surface.

The actions should be linked together and rhythmical, with uniform and gentle exertion of force.

SPECIFIC OPERATION

- **Three-finger squeezing.** Squeeze using the thumb in opposition to the index and middle fingers. (Fig. 35)

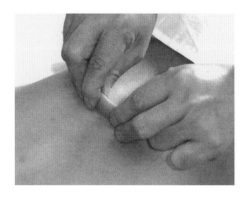

Fig. 35 Three-finger squeezing

- **Five-finger squeezing.** Squeeze using the thumb in opposition to the other four fingers. (Fig. 36)

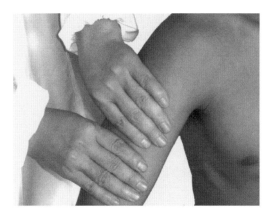

Fig. 36 Five-finger squeezing

Cautions

Movement along the surface of the body should be done slowly; avoid dragging on or jumping along the skin.

Clinical Application

Squeezing provides gentle stimulation and is a common relaxing manipulation. It is usually used on the nape of the neck and limbs, and is often combined with other manipulations to treat disease patterns such as muscle soreness, wind and damp impediment pain, headache and dizziness.

5. Grasping

The thumb pad is used in opposition to the pads of the index and middle fingers (or other four fingers) to perform repeated grasp and release pinching-lifting manipulations. (Fig. 37–38)

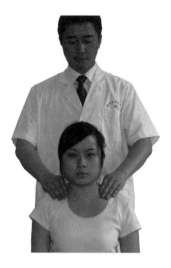

Fig. 37 Five-finger grasping

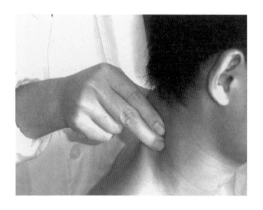

Fig. 38 Three-finger grasping

Movement Principles

POSTURE

The shoulders should be relaxed, the wrists should be agile and the fingers should extend naturally.

BASIC MOVEMENT

Use the thumb in opposition to the other four fingers to firmly grasp the muscle and skin of a certain area, and then gradually increase the pressure while lifting the tissue. The grasping and lifting should continuously alternate between light and heavy.

The exertion of force should continuously and rhythmically flow from light to heavy then back again.

The grasping manipulation may be followed by kneading to relieve discomfort.

Cautions

Avoid digging into the skin with the tips of the fingers.
When lifting, avoid rubbing the skin.

Clinical Application

Grasping provides a relatively strong stimulation, and is a commonly-used treatment and relaxation manipulation. It is appropriate for use on the nape of the neck, shoulders and limbs, and is applied in the treatment of disease patterns such as headache, common cold, muscle soreness and numbness of the limbs.

6. Plucking

In this manipulation the finger pads are placed on certain acupoints or areas and, using moderate strength, perform a one-way or back-and-forth plucking motion perpendicular to the muscle fibres. It is also called collateral plucking, spring plucking and finger plucking. (Fig. 39–42)

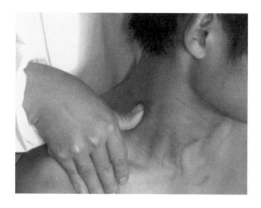

Fig. 39 Single-thumb plucking

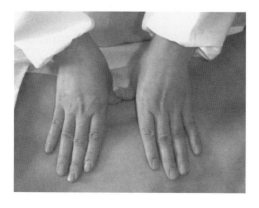

Fig. 40 Stacked-thumb plucking

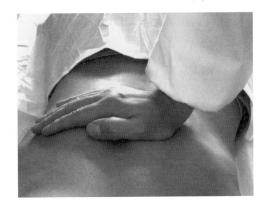

Fig. 41 Palm-base plucking

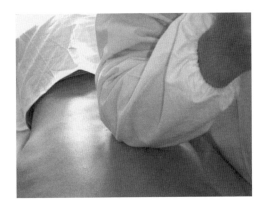

Fig. 42 Elbow plucking

Movement Principles

The downward pressure should not be heavy; take care that it does not exceed what the recipient can tolerate.

Plucking should be done perpendicular to the muscle fibre; if the muscle fibre runs vertically the plucking is done horizontally, and if the muscle fibre runs horizontally the plucking is done vertically.

During plucking the muscle fibres should be moved together. The force used should start light and become heavier, and should penetrate deeply, producing sensations of soreness, pain, distension and numbness.

Cautions

Rubbing on the surface of the skin should be avoided.

This manipulation may not be used in the acute period of soft tissue injury.

Clinical Application

Plucking provides strong stimulation and has the effects of arresting spasm, relieving pain and releasing adhesion. It is a common treatment manipulation, and is primarily applied to the muscles, tendons and fascia of the neck, shoulders, upper and lower back and limbs. It is commonly used in the treatment of localized soft tissue adhesion.

7. Finger Twisting

The thumb and index finger pads are used in opposition to each other to grip then rapidly twist and knead a specific portion of the limbs. (Fig. 43)

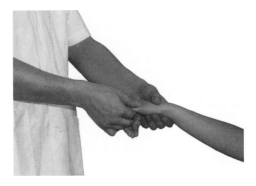

Fig. 43A

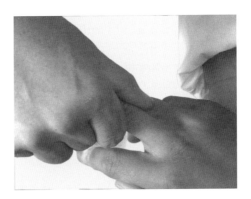

Fig. 43B

Fig. 43 Finger twisting

Movement Principles

POSTURE

Relax the shoulder, elbow and wrist joints.

BASIC MOVEMENT

The fingers press towards each other and twist in a circular fashion as if twisting up a thread.

The movements should be rapid and continuous, but the movement along the treatment area should be slow.

Cautions

The amount of force used by the fingers to press towards each other should be neither too tight nor too loose.

Clinical Application

Finger-twisting provides relatively light stimulation and is one of the smallest Tuina manipulations. This manipulation is primarily applied to the small joints of the four limbs, especially the interphalangeal joints of the fingers. It is used in the treatment of sprain or functional impairment of the fingers or toes.

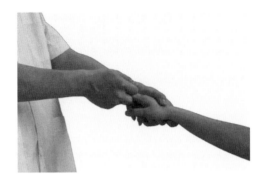

Fig. 44A

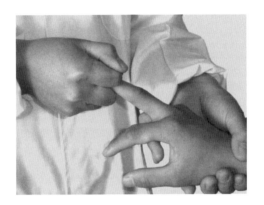

Fig. 44B

Fig. 44 Sliding

8. Sliding

In this manipulation the index and middle fingers are flexed and used to tightly grasp a single finger or toe then slide quickly (while maintaining pressure) from the base to the tip. (Fig. 44)

Movement Principles

While performing the manipulation the wrist should be relaxed and the index and middle fingers of the other hand should be flexed into a 'clamp' shape.

Sliding should be done quickly and the manipulations should be agile, gentle and connected.

Cautions

This manipulation should not be repeated too many times; on average it is performed 3 to 5 times per digit.

Do not use in cases of obvious swelling, fracture, or skin injury of the fingers or toes.

Clinical Application

Sliding provides a moderate level of stimulation, and is a small manipulation that is used to assist with treatment. It is primarily applicable to the small joints of the limbs, and is often combined with finger twisting in the treatment of pain, numbness and functional impairment of the small joints of the limbs.

CHAPTER **6**

Striking Manipulations

The practitioner uses their fingers, palms, fists or special tools to rhythmically strike the surface of the body. This category includes patting and striking.

1. Patting

The practitioner uses their finger pads or empty palms to pat on the surface of the recipient's body. (Fig. 45)

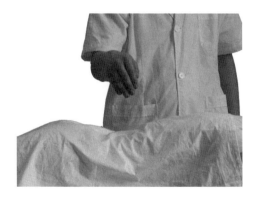

Fig. 45 Patting

Movement Principles

POSTURE

Breathe naturally and relax the shoulders, elbows and wrists. When patting, generate force from the hand and wrist. The movements should be dexterous, springy and rhythmic, and should start light and get heavier.

SPECIFIC OPERATION

- **Finger-pad patting.** The index, middle, ring and little fingers are held together and the finger pads are used to pat on the treatment area. (Fig. 46–47)

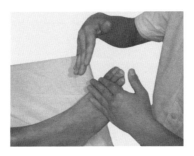

Fig. 46 Finger-pad patting

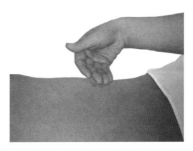

Fig. 47 Finger-back patting

- **Palm patting.** With the fingers held together naturally and the knuckles slightly flexed, the hollow palm is used to pat rhythmically and stably on the surface of the body. (Fig. 48)

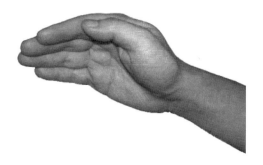

Fig. 48A Hollow palm

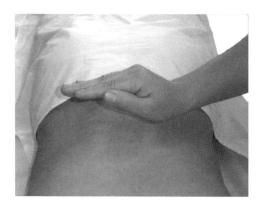

Fig. 48B Hollow palm

Fig. 48 Palm patting

Cautions

The wrist should not be too stiff.

Do not strike the treatment area too forcefully.

Clinical Application

The stimulation provided by patting can be light or heavy, and it is often used as a finishing manipulation at the end of a treatment session. It is appropriate for use on the shoulders, upper back, lower back, buttocks and lower limbs, and has the functions of relieving exhaustion and relaxing the limbs.

2. Striking

The practitioner uses the back of the fist, the base of the palm, the *little fish side* (hypothenar eminence) of the palm, the fingertips or a mulberry wood stick to strike a certain area or acupoint.

Movement Principles

The striking is performed quickly, briefly and gently yet firmly, and the frequency is uniform and rhythmic.

SPECIFIC OPERATION

- **Fingertip striking.** The fingertips are used to lightly rain down strikes on the surface of the body.

- **Fist striking.** The movement of the arm drives a single hollow fist or both fists to strike rhythmically down on the treatment area. (Fig. 49)

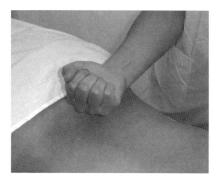

Fig. 49 Fist striking

- **Palm-base striking.** The fingers are separated and slightly flexed and the base of the palm is used to strike on the treatment area. (Fig. 50)

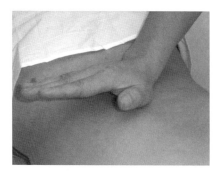

Fig. 50 Palm-base striking

- **Palm-side striking.** With the fingers extended naturally and the wrist flexed slightly backward, the *small fish side* (hypothenar eminence) of one or both hands are used to strike on the body surface. (Fig. 51)

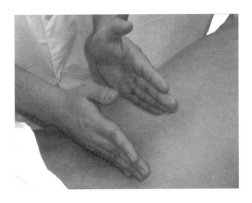

Fig. 51A Single palm-side striking

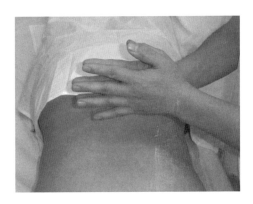

Fig. 51B Double palm-side striking

Fig. 51 Palm-side striking

Cautions

At the beginning of the operation the force used should be light; violent force is prohibited.

When striking, the period of contact with the body surface should be brief, and during that moment of contact one should not drag or pull on the skin.

Clinical Application

Striking provides moderate stimulation, and is often used at the end of a treatment session. Fingertip striking is usually applied to the head, face, chest and abdomen; fist striking is usually used on areas like the lower and upper back; palm-base striking is usually used on the top of the head, lower back, buttocks and limbs; palm-side striking is used on the upper and lower back and the limbs; and stick striking is used on the top of the head, upper and lower back and limbs.

CHAPTER 7

Joint Manipulation Techniques

The techniques in this category involve passive manipulation of the recipient's joints by the practitioner. This includes rotating, thrusting and counter-traction.

1. Rotating

The practitioner moves the joint receiving treatment in a circular motion.

Movement Principles

The practitioner grasps the proximal end of the joint receiving treatment to stabilize the recipient's body. The other hand grasps the distal end of the joint in order to move the joint.

Rotating motions should be slow, and the range of rotation should start small and gradually increase. Stay within the limit of the joint's normal physiological range or within the recipient's tolerable range.

Generally speaking rotation is done half in a clockwise direction and half counter-clockwise.

SPECIFIC OPERATION

- **Neck rotating.** With the recipient sitting, support the back of the recipient's head with one hand and support their lower jaw with the other. Use both hands in coordination to rotate their head to the left and right. (Fig. 52)

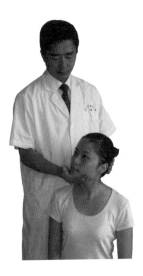

Fig. 52 Neck rotating

- **Shoulder rotating.** Includes shoulder rotating (holding elbow), shoulder rotating (holding hand), shoulder rotating (holding arm) and shoulder rotating (large range).

○ *Shoulder rotating (holding elbow).* With the recipient sitting, press one hand on their shoulder and support their elbow joint with the other hand. Perform clockwise and counter-clockwise rotations. (Fig. 53)

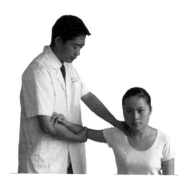

Fig. 53 Shoulder rotating (holding elbow)

○ *Shoulder rotating (holding hand).* With the recipient sitting, press one hand on their shoulder and grasp their hand with the other. Perform clockwise and counter-clockwise rotations. (Fig. 54)

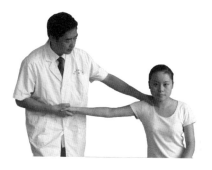

Fig. 54 Shoulder rotating (holding hand)

○ *Shoulder rotating (holding arm).* With the recipient sitting, press one hand on their shoulder and grasp their upper arm with the other. Perform clockwise and counter-clockwise rotations. (Fig. 55)

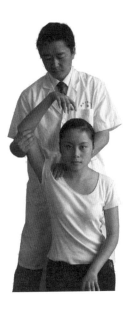

Fig. 55 Shoulder rotating (holding arm)

○ *Shoulder rotating (large range).* With the recipient sitting, stand to one side and clasp their wrist between both hands. Use one hand to grasp their wrist, rotate, turn over, then grasp the wrist again. With the other hand perform pushing and extension of the shoulder joint. The movement of both hands should be coordinated. (Fig. 56)

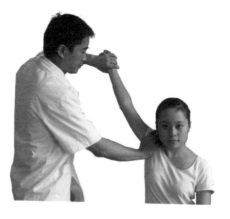

Fig. 56 Shoulder rotating (large range)

- **Elbow rotating.** With one hand holding the recipient's elbow and the other hand holding their wrist, perform circular movements with their elbow in a flexed position. (Fig. 57)

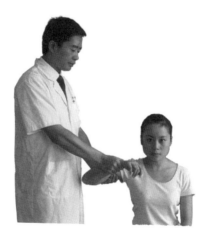

Fig. 57 Elbow rotating

- **Wrist rotating.** With one hand holding the recipient's wrist and the other hand holding their fingers (with the exception of the thumb), rotate the wrist joint. (Fig. 58)

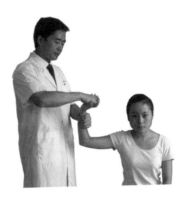

Fig. 58 Wrist rotating

- **Hip rotating.** With the recipient lying face up, flex the recipient's hip and knee. Hold their heel with one hand and place the other hand on top of the knee joint. Perform circular rotating motions of the hip joint. (Fig. 59)

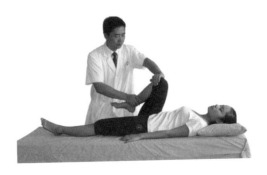

Fig. 59 Hip rotating

- **Knee rotating.** With the recipient lying face down, stand to one side, press one hand down on the upper part of the popliteal fossa (inside of the knee joint), then perform circular rotating motions while holding their ankle with the other. (Fig. 60)

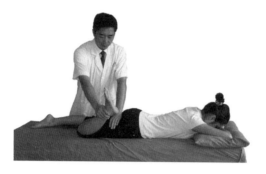

Fig. 60 Knee rotating

- **Ankle rotating.** Grasp the recipient's heel with one hand and hold the base of the foot with the other hand, then rotate the ankle joint. (Fig. 61)

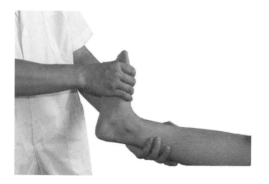

Fig. 61 Ankle rotating

Cautions

The force and speed of the rotation should be even and consistent.

Do not rotate other joints at the same time.

Clinical Application

The emphasis of this manipulation is on moving the joints, and it is a passive guided manipulation. It has the effect of improving the movement function of the joints. This manipulation can be applied to the cervical spine, waist and joints of the limbs. It is used in the treatment of cervical spine pathology, periarthritis of the shoulder, joint rigidity and stiffness, difficulty in extension and flexion, and dyskinesia.

2. Thrusting

Thrusting refers to a manipulation that involves using both hands to suddenly exert force in the same or opposite directions to extend, flex or rotate a joint.

Movement Principles

One of the practitioner's hands acts upon the proximal end of the recipient's joint, and the other acts upon the distal end of the joint.

Begin by performing passive extension, flexion and rotation of the recipient's joint.

Bring the joint to the point of elastic resistance (point of pain).

Next perform a sudden controlled thrust to increase the range.

The final thrusting movement should be brief and rapid. The expression of force should be precise and certain, performed at the right moment, and released immediately.

The thrusting should be performed within the joint's physiological range and limited by the recipient's level of toleration.

SPECIFIC OPERATION

- **Neck thrusting.** Includes inclined neck thrusting and fixed bent neck thrusting.

  ○ *Inclined neck thrusting.* The recipient sits up straight with their head slightly bent forward. With one hand supporting the lower back of their head and the other hand supporting the lower jaw on the opposite side, rotate the head to one side as far as it will go, then thrust with both hands rotating in opposite directions. (Fig. 62)

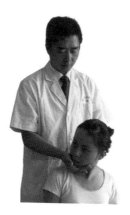

Fig. 62 Inclined neck thrusting

○ *Fixed bent neck thrusting.* With the recipient sitting upright, use one hand to support their lower jaw and press the thumb of the other hand on the side of the cervical spinous processes. At the same time rotate their head towards the affected side to the greatest extent possible, then perform a rapid thrust. (Fig. 63)

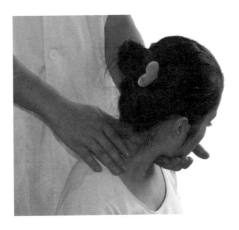

Fig. 63 Fixed bent neck thrusting

• **Chest and back thrusting.** Includes chest traction thrusting and thoracic spine counter-force thrusting.

○ *Chest traction thrusting.* The recipient sits up straight, interlaces their fingers, and places their hands behind their neck. Hold the recipient's elbows with your hands and place one knee at their back. Ask the recipient to bend forward and backward while breathing deeply and perform thrusting to stretch and expand the chest. (Fig. 64)

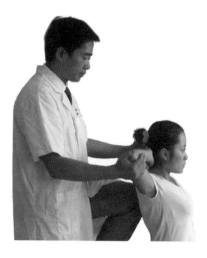

Fig. 64 Chest and back thrusting

○ *Thoracic spine counter-force thrusting.* The recipient sits up straight, interlaces their fingers and places their hands behind their neck. While standing behind the recipient insert one hand in front of each of their upper arms and behind their forearms to grip each arm above the wrist. At the same time place one knee on their spine. Ask the recipient to lean forward slightly and use both hands to thrust upward and backward. (Fig. 65)

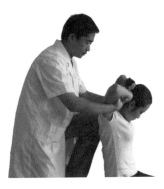

Fig. 65   Thoracic spine counter-force thrusting

- **Waist thrusting.** Includes inclined waist thrusting, waist (rotating) thrusting and backward extension waist thrusting.

    o   *Inclined waist thrusting.* With the recipient lying on one side, place one hand on the front of their shoulder and the other hand on their buttock area (or place one hand on the back of their shoulder and the other hand on the upper anterior iliac spine). Rotate the waist as far as possible, then thrust with both hands moving in opposite directions. (Fig. 66)

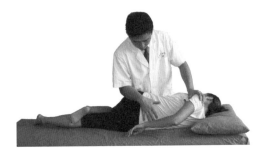

Fig. 66   Inclined waist thrusting

○   *Waist (rotating) thrusting*

•   Straight waist (rotating) thrusting. With the recipient sitting up straight, use the legs to stabilize the recipient's lower limbs while standing to one side. Place one hand on the back of the shoulder closest to you and insert the other hand under their other armpit and around to the front to hold the front of their shoulder. Thrust the hands in opposite directions to perform the manipulation. (Fig. 67)

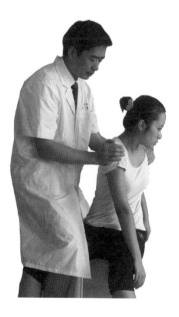

Fig. 67 Straight waist (rotating) thrusting

- Bent waist (rotating) thrusting. The recipient sits and bends forward as far as is necessary. An assistant helps to hold down the recipient's lower limbs and pelvis. Press one thumb on the spinous process of the vertebra receiving the manipulation (when turning left use the right hand) and hook the other hand around the back of the recipient's neck (when turning left use the left hand). With the recipient bent forward, turn their waist towards the affected side. When it is turned as far as possible, thrust by pressing towards the healthy side with the thumb and turning the upper body in the other direction with your other hand. (Fig. 68)

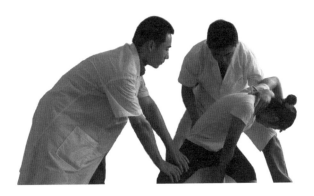

Fig. 68 Bent waist (rotating) thrusting

○ *Backward extension waist thrusting.* With the recipient lying face down, place one hand under the recipient's knees and slowly raise them up. Press firmly on the affected area of the lower back with the other hand, and when the waist is extended as far as possible thrust with both hands in opposite directions. (Fig. 69)

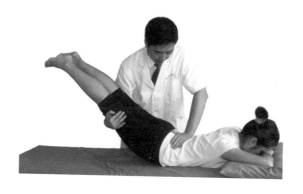

Fig. 69 Backward extension waist thrusting

- **Shoulder thrusting.** Includes shoulder thrusting (adduct), shoulder thrusting (abduct), backward extension shoulder thrusting and vertical shoulder thrusting.

○ *Shoulder thrusting (adduct).* The recipient sits with their elbow flexed and held in front of their chest. Stand behind the recipient and press your body against their back to stabilize their torso. With the arm on the same side of the recipient's flexed arm, press down on their shoulder and grip their elbow with the other hand. Adduct the shoulder joint until you meet resistance, then quickly and resolutely thrust in a controlled fashion. (Fig. 70)

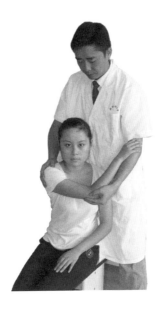

Fig. 70 Shoulder thrusting (adduct)

○ *Shoulder thrusting (abduct).* With the recipient sitting upright, interlace your fingers and place them on the shoulder to clasp the front and back of the shoulder joint. At the same time, rest the recipient's upper arm on your forearm. Extend and open the shoulder joint until resistance is felt, then thrust by pressing down with the hands and lifting with the forearm to abduct the shoulder joint. (Fig. 71)

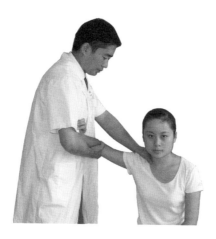

Fig. 71 Shoulder thrusting (abduct)

○ *Backward extension shoulder thrusting.* The recipient sits or lies on their side. Press one hand on the back of their shoulder and hold their arm with the other hand. Extend the arm backward then lift until it meets resistance and perform a small amplitude upward thrust. The other hand should be stabilizing the shoulder joint and torso. (Fig. 72)

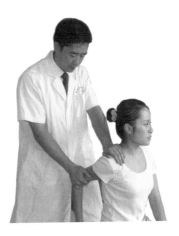

Fig. 72 Backward extension shoulder thrusting

○ *Vertical shoulder thrusting.* The recipient sits with their arms hanging down freely. Stand behind the recipient and use one arm to grip the recipient's arm above the elbow, then slowly lift the arm to the front or to the side to 120–140°. Grip the recipient's upper or lower arm with the other arm and use both hands to gradually apply traction upward on the arm until it meets resistance. Extend the range by performing a small and controlled upward thrust. (Fig. 73)

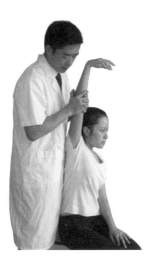

Fig. 73 Vertical shoulder thrusting

- **Elbow thrusting.** The recipient sits or lies face up. Hold the back of the elbow joint with one hand and grip the wrist with the other hand. Flex and extend the elbow joint repeatedly, then when the joint is extended as far as possible thrust with both hands (the hand holding the elbow stabilizes the elbow joint). (Fig. 74)

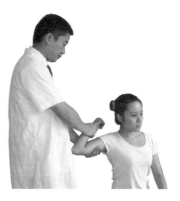

Fig. 74 Elbow thrusting

• **Wrist thrusting.** The recipient sits or lies face up. Hold the recipient's arm above the wrist with one hand, and hold their palm or fingers with the other hand (interlace the fingers). First apply traction on the wrist joint, then thrust. Thrust up and down to flex and extend the joint and thrust to the left and right to abduct and adduct the joint. The main manipulations are flexing and extending. (Fig. 75)

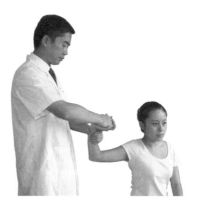

Fig. 75 Wrist thrusting

- **Hip thrusting.** The recipient lies face up with their hip and knee joint flexed. Hold their heel with one hand while supporting their knee with the other hand and rotate the hip joint. Alternately extend and flex the hip joint 4 to 5 times, then flex the hip joint until resistance is felt and thrust using both hands. Other variations include '#4' thrusting, straight leg thrusting and backward extension thrusting. (Fig. 76)

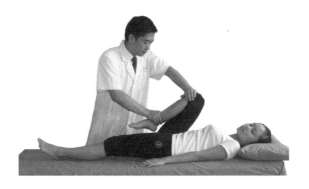

Fig. 76 Hip thrusting

- **Knee thrusting.** The recipient sits or lies face up. Press down on the back of the knee joint with one hand and grip the ankle with the other hand. Flex and extend the knee joint repeatedly, then when the joint is flexed as far as possible perform a fast large-range thrust. (Fig. 77)

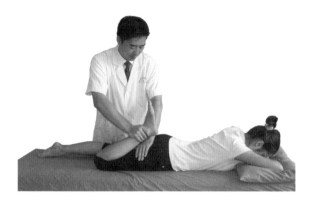

Fig. 77 Knee thrusting

• **Ankle thrusting.** The recipient lies face up or face down. Hold their heel with one hand and hold the sole of their foot with the other hand. First pull out on the ankle joint, then perform dorsiflex and plantar flexing to thrust the ankle. Two hands may be used at the same time. (Fig. 78)

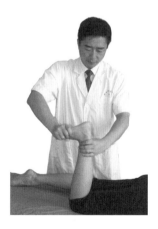

Fig. 78 Ankle thrusting

Cautions

Take care not to exceed the joint's normal physiological range.

It is not necessary to 'crack' the joint every time.

This manipulation is not to be used in the case of osteoarticular tuberculosis, bone tumors, severe joint degeneration or for patients with signs of spinal cord compression.

Clinical Application

Thrusting is a regulating manipulation that can correct dislocation and release soft tissue adhesion. This manipulation can be applied to joints of the neck, chest, waist, limbs, etc. It is used in the treatment of dislocation of the cervical, thoracic and lumbar vertebra and coccyx, as well as functional joint disorder of the limbs.

3. Counter-Traction

The practitioner uses counter-strength to pull and stretch the recipient's joints or limbs.

Movement Principles

The movements should be steady and gentle.

The force should be even and continuous. It should start small and gradually increase.

The force and direction of counter-traction must be appropriate for the area of treatment.

SPECIFIC OPERATION

- **Head and neck counter-traction**

    1. With the recipient sitting, stand directly behind them. Place both thumbs under the recipient's occiput while clasping their lower jaw with the base of each palm to provide support, then lift upward with both hands to provide upward traction. (Fig. 79)

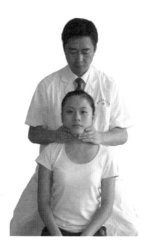

Fig. 79 Head and neck counter-traction (1)

    2. With the recipient sitting, place one hand at the back of the recipient's occiput and wrap the other elbow around their lower jaw with the same hand supporting their temple. Use both hands at the same time to provide upward traction. (Fig. 80)

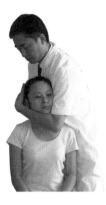

Fig. 80 Head and neck counter-traction (2)

3. The recipient lies face up with their head and neck extending over the edge of the bed. Sit behind the recipient's head. Cradle the recipient's lower jaw with one elbow and place the other hand under the recipient's occiput and pull with both hands to provide traction. During this process the recipient's head should be kept level or tilted slightly forward. Rotating movements may also be performed while stretching the cervical vertebrae. (Fig. 81)

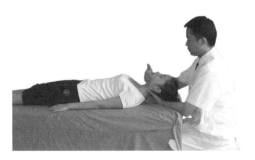

Fig. 81 Head and neck counter-traction (3)

- **Shoulder counter-traction**

    1. The recipient sits on a low stool and relaxes their upper limbs. Stand behind and off to one side of the recipient and use both hands to hold their elbow and wrist and gradually lift the arm upward. The recipient can lean in the opposite direction to resist the pull or an assistant can support their body. (Fig. 82)

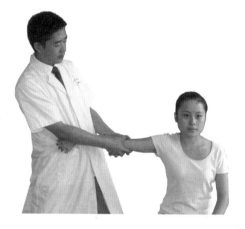

Fig. 82 Shoulder counter-traction (1)

    2. With the recipient seated, place one knee in their armpit and pull down on their arm with both hands gripping their wrist. (Fig. 83)

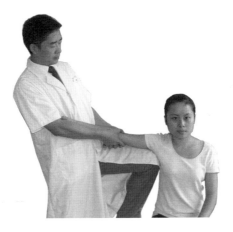

Fig. 83 Shoulder counter-traction (2)

- **Elbow counter-traction.** Use both hands to grip the recipient's wrist area. The assistant uses both hands to grip the recipient's upper arm. The two practitioners use opposing force to perform counter-traction of the elbow joint. (Fig. 84)

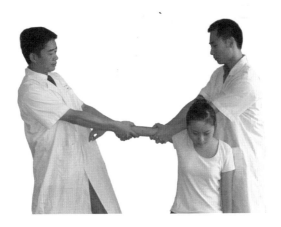

Fig. 84 Elbow counter-traction

- **Finger (or toe) counter-traction.** With one hand holding the distal end of the recipient's finger and the other hand holding the proximal end, use opposing force with each hand to perform counter-traction on the finger joints. (The same technique can be applied to the toe.) (Fig. 85)

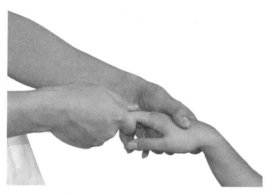

Fig. 85 Finger counter-traction

- **Waist counter-traction.** The recipient lies face down and holds onto the edge of the bed tightly with both hands. Alternately the recipient lies face up and an assistant holds their armpits to support their body. Grasp each of the recipient's legs above the ankles, and then gradually pull on their legs to perform counter-traction on the joints of the waist. (Fig. 86)

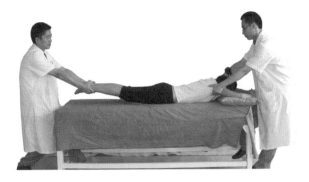

Fig. 86 Waist counter-traction

- **Ankle counter-traction.** With the recipient lying face up or sitting on the bed, hold one of the recipient's legs above the ankle with one hand and hold the sole of their foot with the other hand. Use opposing force with both hands to perform counter-traction on the ankle joint. (Fig. 87)

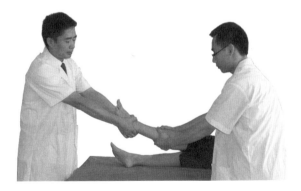

Fig. 87 Ankle counter-traction

Cautions

When performing counter-traction sudden or abrupt use of force is prohibited.

Clinical Application

This manipulation is often used in the treatment of displaced tendons and joint dislocation. It has the effects of rectifying dislocation, correcting deformation, enlarging joint space and lessening compression stimulation.